YOUR KNOWLEDGE HAS VALUE

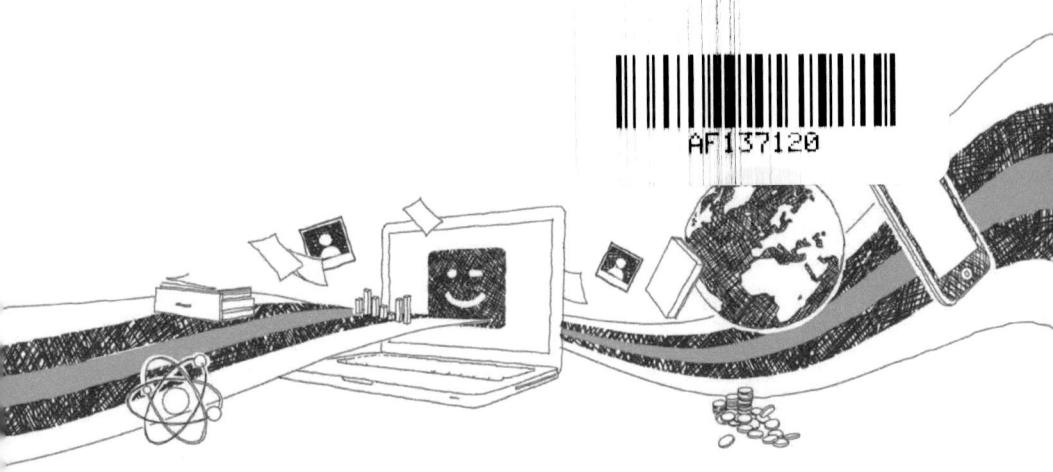
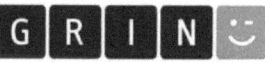

Bibliographic information published by the German National Library:

The German National Library lists this publication in the National Bibliography; detailed bibliographic data are available on the Internet at http://dnb.dnb.de .

Imprint:

Copyright © 2018 GRIN Verlag
Print and binding: Books on Demand GmbH, Norderstedt Germany
ISBN: 9783346060822

This book at GRIN:

https://www.grin.com/document/505421

Daniela Hettich

Cancer in adolescents. Communication and information provision at the diagnostic consultation

The effect on participation in treatment decision-making. An extended literature review

GRIN Verlag

GRIN - Your knowledge has value

Since its foundation in 1998, GRIN has specialized in publishing academic texts by students, college teachers and other academics as e-book and printed book. The website www.grin.com is an ideal platform for presenting term papers, final papers, scientific essays, dissertations and specialist books.

Visit us on the internet:

http://www.grin.com/

http://www.facebook.com/grincom

http://www.twitter.com/grin_com

Literature Review Research Project

by
Daniela Elisabeth Hettich

Published October 2019

Cancer in adolescents: How do communication and information provision at the diagnostic consultation affect the adolescent's participation in treatment decision-making? An extended review of the literature.

"To speak is to occupy the world" from William Hanks, cited in Clemente (2015, p.6)

Table of Contents

Abbreviations and Glossary

AAP	American Academy of Pediatrics
AYA	Adolescents and young adults
HCPs	Health care professionals
NHS	National health service
SDM	Shared decision-making
SIOP	International society of paediatric oncology
	(Société international d'oncologie péediatrique)
TCT	Teenage Cancer Trust
TM	Therapeutic misconception
UNCRC	United Nations Convention of the Rights of the Child (1989)

Assent

Assent signifies agreement and demonstrates the child's involvement in decision-making and is required by the Declaration of Helsinki. In the UK the Royal College of Paediatrics and Child Heath recommends obtaining assent from the age of seven, as does the American Academy of Pediatrics.

Consent

Consent gives legal permission for treatment to be carried out or participation in research. In Scotland 16-year-olds are considered old enough to make their own decisions without their parents. In England and Wales 16 and 17-year-olds can provide consent but so can their parents.

Dissent

The refusal of treatment or trial participation. EU and UK guidelines suggest that a minor's wishes and objections be seriously taken into consideration.

Oncology

A field of medicine specializing in the diagnosis and treatment of cancer.

Prognosis

In the context of this review means prediction of survival chances.

Therapeutic misconception

An ethical issue, where failure to understand the difference between ordinary treatment and clinical research may result in trial participation in the belief that they might benefit from the findings, rather than a benefit gained for future patients.

Survivor

In the field of cancer treatment, a survivor is a broad term generally covering the time span from cancer diagnosis until the patient's death.

Terminology

Due to the use of the different terms used in the literature to cover the age range from 12 to 20, and unless specifically used to differentiate, the terms teenager, young person, and sometimes children refer to an adolescent. The terms physician, clinician and oncologist are interchangeable and refer to the consulting doctor. The terms parents and guardians are also used interchangeably.

Age range

The chronological age range for the adolescents referred to in this review is extrapolated to range from 12 up to 20 years, which is above the legal age of adulthood but included because specific teenage cancer units treat patients up to their 20th birthday, upon which they transition to adult units.

Abstract

The purpose of this literature review is to examine the question, 'How do communication and information provision of the cancer diagnosis affect the adolescents' participation in treatment decision-making?'. To find evidence to answer this question, a literature search was conducted using the databases available to me through the Open University library.

It was found that despite the recognition of the importance of adequate information provision, adolescent cancer patients and their caregivers feel that they are not adequately informed by physicians who use regulated communication to control information provision. For cancer survivors, insufficient information provision at diagnosis has left them with knowledge gaps in their medical history. For the newly diagnosed patient inadequate information provision limits their understanding of the illness, weakening their ability to participate in their treatment decision-making. Parental culture and the involvement of the adolescent in decision-making in the family unit prior to illness affect how decision-making is approached in the oncological setting. In the triadic decision-making constellation, parents act as barriers to adolescent involvement by shielding their children from negative findings and taking over responsibility in decision-making. The nature of the illness, treatment protocols and organizational constraints further constrain adolescents' activity in decision-making. Whilst adolescents want to be informed, their participatory behaviour is varied ranging from being present during consultation to autonomous decision-making.

The main implication for health-care professionals is that the best interests of the adolescent are served if their information and participation preferences are sought prior to the first consultation upon which, ideally, a more collaborative and tailored approach could be applied. In furtherance to this, research on adolescent information preferences and full disclosure at diagnosis should be conducted, as presently the emphasis is still on containment and protectionism.

Keywords: Cancer, paediatric (pediatric) oncology, adolescent, young person, communication, information, diagnosis, shared decision-making.

Introduction

Adolescents are at a crossroads between childhood and adulthood; a time of change, uncertainty and maturity. A cancer diagnosis presents more uncertainty and affects how they view themselves in relation to their family and peers. Out of the instinct to protect, adolescents are not always provided with full information about their disease or treatment consequences, despite the fact that they will be involved in decision-making regarding their treatment and possible participation in clinical trials. Research on children's participation in decision-making is growing but there is limited research into the adolescents' role especially in cancer treatment. This review seeks to contribute to the field by examining how communication and information provision at the diagnostic consultation affect adolescent participation in treatment decision-making.

Because of the rarity of the illness, the relative new field and the sensitive nature of research, the studies mostly consist of small cohorts of participants. The sources used stem mainly from a variety of studies within clinical settings, with scientific papers and texts, as well as encyclopaedias used for clarification of terms or to underscore theory. Whilst adolescents are central for this review, perspectives from parents and physicians are also included. Findings from similar research for adult cancer patients on communication and decision-making are excluded because their relevance rests outside of this literature review.

The structure of the review body is broken down into five sections. Adolescent cancer incidence is the first, followed by a description of the diagnostic consultation in the second. The third section discusses the themes of communication, information-sharing and the consequences of unmet information needs in the clinical setting. In section four, legislation and the shared decision-making framework are outlined. Section five examines how the three participants, namely adolescent patient, parent and physician interact and their respective role in the decision-making triad. Further, the challenges arising from this constellation are examined and discussed.

Directly after the review body, a critical analysis of the research study findings follows. The emergent themes and arguments are discussed here and conclude with the argument that the adolescent patient's needs and rights to be heard are not sufficiently met. The links to practice and its implications follow on from this together with recommendations for policy.

The conclusion summarises the main points and regarding communication and information provision, finds that adolescents want to be fully informed, but parents and physicians attempt to shield them by controlling the data provided. The suggestion for research to be continued in this area, specifically on adolescent preferences for information provision and full disclosure at diagnosis is made. Whilst adolescent participation in decision-making is constrained by the nature of the illness and the attitudes of health care professionals and parents, provision for involvement in minor decisions is made. As the burden of cancer treatment decision-making is hard to carry alone, adolescents seek support from their parents.

Cancer Incidence in Adolescents

Cancer is a life-threatening and in some cases a life-limiting disease with complex and invasive treatment schedules. Despite the progress made in curing some cancers, it continues to remain the most common cause of death through illness in adolescents and young adults (AYAs) in high-income countries (Bleyer et al., 2017). Statistical information on incidence is provided in Appendix A. The increasing frequency has seen a new, specific group of cancer patients emerge, situated between paediatric and adult care, facing lower cure rates and with their own psychosocial and cultural needs (Thompson et al., 2013).

A cancer diagnosis has an impact at any stage in life, but when it affects adolescents, who are going through a time of transformation, both physically and developmentally, it can be devastating. The significance on further growth and maturation is considerable (Magni et al., 2015). Adolescents are at a defining intersection of their development, namely the area between striving for individuation, whilst still being financially and emotionally dependent. A cancer diagnosis increases this dependency. As their future becomes less certain and their social activities curtailed, the natural process of independence becomes more difficult (Phillips-Salami et al., 2014). Adolescents experience a loss of normalcy (Brand et al., 2017; Magni et al., 2015). Hair loss, unwanted weight loss or gain and mutilating surgery can all become major issues especially at a time when young people are most concerned about self-image. Cancer also increases isolation, crucially at a time when peers and society are most important to the psychological well-being of adolescents. Schooling and education suffer through erratic attendance adding to their concerns (Teenage Cancer Trust, 2016). These factors place the adolescent cancer patient in an emotionally vulnerable position. As adolescents also tend to express negative emotions more strongly than children (Korsvold et al., 2016a) the communication of their cancer diagnosis may be affected by this.

The Diagnostic Consultation

The formal diagnosis often follows a period of apprehension, suspicion and guessing, often involving misdiagnosis; a time when the adolescent and family are already feeling vulnerable and emotionally drained (Phillips et al., 2017). Survivors recount their diagnosis experience as a 'terrorist attack' (Phillips et al., 2017, p. 3) underscoring the importance of the manner, in which the diagnosis is communicated. Kessel et al. (2013) find that it affects how the patient and their family react to the news and Korsvold et al. (2016b) suggest that there may be a link between how diagnosis is delivered with the levels of stress, anxiety and general satisfaction experienced in the patient's ensuing healthcare. The diagnostic consultation is an extremely challenging situation where a balance needs to be found between conveying realistic facts, retaining hope and aiming to regulate strong emotions (Magni et al., 2015). It is generally agreed that the setting for disclosure is in a quiet, private setting and that the information provided and gathered should be clearly communicated as these will inform decision-making in treatment and therapy (Wiering et al., 2016).

The adolescent cancer patient will be involved in decisions regarding different treatment therapies which may include chemotherapy, radiotherapy, surgery or amputation. Ideally, during the diagnostic consultation, the patient is told of their disease; name; stage; causation; prognosis and treatment. In practice however, often neither a full diagnosis nor adequate information is provided for the patient to make informed decisions (Clemente, 2015). Physicians may choose to avoid talking about prognosis out of concern of the emotional impact and if asked, by replying obscurely or in unduly optimistic terms (Mack and Joffe, 2014) or even by attacking perceived negative questions (Clement, 2015).

Treatment options may be limited as many cancers, such as bone cancer, only use evidence-based treatment protocols (Clemente, 2007). If multiple treatment options exist, they can be presented with a discussion of the advantages and disadvantages of the different courses of action (Kessel et al., 2013). An explanation of the treatment, drugs, their administration and side effects should be provided. The short-term adverse effects, such as nausea, hair loss, and fatigue need to be conveyed to prepare patients and their families to deal with the immediate consequences. Both radiotherapy and chemotherapy can cause infertility and thus decisions concerning fertility preservation, for example semen cryopreservation or embryo-freezing need to be made before treatment begins. Gender and age determine the likelihood of referral to a fertility clinic with females and pre-pubescent males the least likely to be adequately informed and referred (Yeomanson et al., 2013). This could be attributed to the lack of technical possibilities in fertility preservation or the professional approach to communication (Yeomanson et al., 2013). Adverse long-term effects of treatment can be serious and life-threatening such as disability, secondary cancers and cardio-pulmonary toxicity. Although physicians believe these should be discussed, there are differing opinions amongst the physicians on what side effects should be disclosed (Olson et al., 2012). A decision regarding participation in clinical trials may be necessary and require full explanation so that in the case of a minor, they can provide their assent or agreement to participation (de Vries et al., 2011). This important decision needs to be made under time and emotional pressure and in order to understand the implications and risks of trials, good communication is crucial (de Vries et al., 2011).

The procedural steps of the diagnostic consultation have been illustrated as has the content. However, there are two notable omissions in this process. The first is the option of palliative care which is rarely communicated at diagnosis if the treatment plan is curative, despite growing evidence of the value it brings when used as a parallel form of treatment (Wiener et al., 2014). Although physicians acknowledge its value when implemented from the beginning, they still tend to delay referral until late into the illness (Twamley et al., 2014). The second omission, which will be addressed further in this review, is the fact that the patient is asked neither about their preferences for how they want to receive information nor how they want to be involved in treatment decision-making.

Communication and Information Sharing

The term 'communication' means to 'make common, share, participate, or impart' (Bosco and Angeleri, 2010). The communication of a cancer diagnosis therefore suggests information sharing and finding commonality in treatment decisions.

Adequate information provision on a patient's health is a moral obligation. The International Society of Pediatric Oncology (SIOP) specifically addresses the importance of providing information in relation to maturity and age when communicating with adolescents and young adults (Magni et al., 2015). In addition to fulfilling ethical requirements, information provision helps adolescents understand their illness, thus providing a way of coping with their uncertain situation (Bahrami et al., 2017). By sharing information with pediatric patients, their fears can be explored and discussed (Wangmo et al., 2017). Additionally, anxiety and depression can be reduced when some of the uncertainty is removed (Bahrami et al., 2017). The concealment of bad news does not provide protection, especially not in the long-term. Mack and Joffe (2014) found that even a poor prognosis can relieve distress and sustain hope if the conversation is honest and supportive. Parents need information so that they can plan their child's care and support them despite the risk of distress it may cause (Ilowite et al., 2017).

Patients and their guardians need to be informed about the difference between therapeutic interventions based on the individual patient's needs and research, which follows protocols dictated by the specific clinical trials (Alderson, 2007). Treatment is diagnostic, preventative, curative or palliative and aims to improve the patient's current well-being. Research tends to benefit future patients (de Vries et al., 2011). Since most treating paediatric oncologists tend to be involved in research there may be an overlap in interests, raising potential ethical issues (Dekking et al, 2015). The distinction and significance this has for an individual's treatment may not be apparent and if patients or guardians are unaware of this, it is known as therapeutic misconception (de Clercq et al., 2017).

Most children and their parents require and value information so that they can actively collaborate with health care providers (HCPs) and participate in decision-making (Wiering et al., 2016). Adolescents value a reciprocal information exchange contributing information about their own lives and health condition (Weaver et al., 2015). Participation increases the family's cooperation in treatment decisions (Kilicarslan-Toruner and Akgun-Citak, 2013) and crucially, adolescent treatment compliance which can otherwise be erratic (Phillips et al., 2017).

Yet, despite these arguments for adequate information provision, physicians still regulate information communication during the consultation by 'filtering' the amount and content according to what they perceive to be relevant and controlling the timing of when it is given, known as 'pacing' (Ruhe et al., 2016b, p. 1150). Clemente (2007) finds that physicians strategically avoid answering difficult questions by giving non-answer responses such as reassurances; not providing a full answer; a contingent answer which is accurate but is linked to a condition and forestalling a question.

Furthermore, hospital culture and the hierarchical structure influence how information is communicated and shared (Wiering et al., 2016). Patients and parents are often dissatisfied with information provided by physicians and the lack of open discussion (Badarau et al., 2015). The terminology used is often euphemistic or ambiguous, for example rather than confirm that the disease is terminal, the physician might formulate this as 'informing the teenagers of test results and the difficulties moving forward.' (Day et al., 2017, p.4). Not everyone understands these nuances and subtexts and if prognosis is not directly addressed, the physician might assume the patient does not want to know because they do not enquire whilst the patient could believe that if it is not mentioned it must not be important (Ruhe et al., 2016b; Back et al. 2005). Of the parents interviewed, Kessel et al. (2013) found that 90% wanted unambiguous language to be used, specifically the term 'cancer' and 92% wanted to know the cure rate. Rost et al. (2017 p. 561) found that parent dissatisfaction with discussions stemmed from physicians' often 'overly optimistic assessment of the prognosis.' Although cancer prognosis can be inaccurate, particularly in paediatric oncology, there are several reasons to provide prognostic information namely; to reduce uncertainty; allow for priority setting; making appropriate treatment choices and forming a trusting relationship with the physician. It also shows respect for the patient and their care-givers (Kessel et al., 2013). Clinicians are reluctant to provide prognostic news because they fear that hope will be negatively impacted (Rost et al., 2017).

Insufficient information provision at diagnosis (Vetsch et al., 2017) has left a significant number of survivors of paediatric cancer with gaps in their medical history such as on treatment toxicities, impacting their future lives (Phillips et al., 2017). When information needs remain unmet, anxiety caused by uncertainty leads to negative health-related quality of life (de Rouen et al., 2015). Adolescents feel strongly about being lied to or having information withheld from them and may withdraw cooperation if they feel they cannot trust the physician to be honest with them (Bahrami et al., 2017). Indeed, Clemente (2007 p.19) found that:

> 'information withholding by clinicians was shown to greatly limit adolescents' ability to participate in the management of their treatment''.

Problematic communication between professionals and adolescents leads to reduced access to relevant information (Essig et al., 2016). If adolescents lack information, they can feel isolated and disassociate themselves from the decision-making process (Bahrami et al., 2017). For a young person to be able to form an opinion, they need access to adequate information (de Clercq et al., 2017), which is crucial to decision-making Alderson (2007). When adolescents do not receive information directly from the physician, they use their parents as information brokers (Young et al., 2003) who then act as intermediaries. They also resort to consulting less reliable sources (Essig et al., 2016), where data can be distressing and confusing (Brand et al., 2017).

When information preferences are assumed, rather than sought, misunderstandings occur. Day et al (2017, p.4) found that physicians believe that they have 'learned to pick up cues from teenagers about the level of information they wish to have' (Day et al. 2017, p.4) through their experience, which differs from a study by Thompson et al. (2013), who find disparity between what is important to adolescents and what HCPs perceive is important. Young people's top priority related to their immediate future, which differs from the expectations of physicians who assume survival to be of top priority. Notably, adequate information provision, necessary for decision-making is listed by AYAs and omitted by HCPs. The full table is included as Appendix B. Assumptions about culture can also impact the information process Bahrami et al. (2017) and Ilowite et al. (2017) find that clinicians underestimate the amount of prognostic information patients require, particularly in the black and Hispanic population. Differing perceptions are also found by Rost et al., (2017) who found that parents feel that their children are more competent to understand diagnosis and prognosis than their physicians do. They also found that whilst parents were dissatisfied with information provision, physicians thought it to be adequate. A case study of the diagnostic consultation related by a patient and their family is included as Appendix C. It illustrates the challenges faced by physicians in managing the expectations they themselves have raised during the diagnostic consultation.

Having argued the case for adequate information provision, it must be noted that not all children want full information but instead prefer to have more control over when and how they receive it (Kelly et al., 2016). And, just as clinicians can withhold poor prognosis from adolescent patients and their care-givers in an effort to protect them, guardians also conceal information from their children (Coyne et al. 2014) and act as gate-keepers to information provision (Bahrami et al., 2017). Parents shield their children by seeking consultations with physicians without the presence of the patient (Wiering et al., 2016), thereby also 'filtering' and 'pacing' the information provided (Ruhe et al., 2016b p. 1150). This coalition building can negatively affect the relationship between the patient and physician (Gabe et al., 2004). If, in an attempt to avoid distress, open communication between parents and adolescent breaks down, it can lead to negative health issues for both parties (Phillips-Salami et al., 2014). Parents' concerns for their child's welfare may override recognition of their growing autonomy and independence (Nuffield, 2015). Stakeholders, for fear of upsetting each other, may not openly communicate or pose controversial questions, enabling a situation where difficult subjects are evaded or avoided and thereby impairing decision-making (Bluebond-Langer et al., 2005). Despite the obvious need for adolescents' involvement in their own health care, their access to information is limited. In the next section the complexity of shared decision-making will be shown to further decreases their ability to participate in treatment decision-making.

Shared Decision-making

The UK government's policy is to make shared decision-making (SDM) part of the NHS treatment plan, requiring that physicians and patients work together in defining and choosing the most appropriate treatment plan for an individual. The SDM model combines the expertise of the physician with the experience and knowledge of the patient, evaluates the medical evidence and balances these with a patient's values, attitudes to risk and their social circumstances and preferences (Coulter and Collins, 2011). Legislation, namely United Nations Convention on the Rights of the Child (UNCRC, 1989) has established the need for children and adolescents to participate in the decision-making process and attempts are made to incorporate these into the framework of the healthcare setting (Wangmo et al., 2017). Being involved in decision-making empowers adolescents to hone their self-management skills, gain back some control and influence their situation (Kelly et al., 2016). It also provides them with recognition and respect; human needs necessary to well-being. As experts of their own illness, experience and values, adolescents can contribute in the decision-making process and generally want to (Kelly et al., 2016). Nevertheless, these preferences vary and in the paediatric oncology context, the circumstances under which adolescents can voice their preferences and participate in decision-making cannot reflect the agency they would have without living with cancer (Brand et al., 2017).

In the context of the UNCRC (1989) the three fundamental principles of provision, protection and participation are combined in the directive of 'best interest' of the child. This is used as the guiding principle in health care but guidance on its implementation in paediatric practice is limited and various challenges occur in its implementation. The directive 'best interest' is open to different interpretations based on family values and sociocultural context (Graham and Fitzgerald, 2010). Parenting style and attitudes towards independence within the family unit influence how adolescents participate in decision-making in the clinical setting (Wangmo et al., 2017). Children want to retain the 'normalcy' of family life and how they have been included or excluded in family decision-making prior to their illness, may affect their participation in this setting (Bluebond-Langer et al., 2005). The SIOP recommend that children are included in decision-making in ways which are appropriate to their developmental stage. But their participation is limited (Coyne et al., 2016) and in the oncological setting, participation ranges from being present at a consultation and receiving information through to treatment decision-making (Ruhe et al. 2016a).

Informed consent is both a legal and moral requirement based on respect for a patient's autonomy (Alderson, 2007). But a consensus on what constitutes competency to consent to clinical research or treatment is still lacking (Hein et al., 2015) and the age at which patients are considered legally competent to make medical decisions varies from country to country, ranging from 12 to 16 years of age (de Clercq et al., 2017). Adolescents generally have the capacity and cognitive reasoning skills to appraise treatment options (Steinberg,2013) but decision-making capacity cannot be judged by age alone since ability matures with time and experience (Unguru, 2011) and severely ill children are often cognitively ahead of their age group as a result (Wangmo et al., 2017). As cancer treatment is aggressive and adolescents surviving the treatment could live with its effects for years, it is crucial that the implications of treatment are understood (de Rouen et al., 2015) and consent (or assent for those not eligible to consent) is given. Article 12 of the UNCRC (1989) specifically requires that HCPs discuss healthcare issues directly with the child and elicit their understanding and opinions (Streuli et al., 2011). Examples of these types of questions are included in Appendix D. Nonetheless, Wiering et al. (2016) found that physicians still tend to inform rather than elicit involvement. They also found that 'in only two out of 43 consultations explicit permission to start treatment was asked', despite legal and ethical requirements Wiering et al. (2016, p. 64). The authors postulate that in order for the child to survive, the treatment is considered necessary and therefore consent is seen as a formality rather than a necessity. Legally, when a child is below the age of consent they will require their guardian to act as a surrogate decision-maker, changing the dyadic decision-making relationship to a triadic one (de Clercq et al., 2017).

Often there is little opportunity for adolescent participation in treatment decision-making as protocol and seriousness of the disease dictate treatment and schedule. These are under the auspices of the physician, especially when the defining factor is cure (Whitney et al. 2006). In their research Kilicarslan-Toruner and Akgun-Citak (2013) found that the decision-making process is rarely a collaboration, but rather the physician's decision. Indeed, de Vries et al. (2010) suggest that physicians believe adolescents to be too emotionally overwhelmed to make treatment decisions. Physicians act as facilitators, and as such can greatly influence communication in the decision-making process. The nature and stage of the illness demand that physicians consult other professionals, thereby widening the decision-making scope but lessening the input or validity of the patient (Day et al., 2017). HCPs identified insufficient time and difficulty in finding the appropriate language to address children as constraining factors in participation (Wangmo et al 2017). Importantly they also list "the fear of losing power by having their views questioned" which puts into question the validity of shared decision-making Wangmo et al. (2017, p.11).

When adolescent patients refuse treatment, paediatric oncologists face a dilemma as they are obliged to work in the best interest of the child, whilst respecting their autonomy (Essig et al., 2017). Researchers find that physicians can more readily accept refusal of cancer treatment if prognosis is poor, even when parents disagree (Talati et al., 2010). In a situation where there is a good chance of cure, the courts can enforce a 17-year old for example to undergo chemotherapy treatment. Conversely, when a 13-year old suffering from chemotherapy induced cardiomyopathy, refused a heart transplant the decision was upheld by the courts in recognition of her life experience and autonomy Olzweski and Goldkind 2018). Thus, not only do age, experience, insight and maturity play a part in decision-making, but the benefits and risks involved also require assessment (Olzweski and Goldkind 2018).

The Triadic Decision-making Constellation

Parents see themselves as communication executives who retain the overview, pose questions, supplement and provide details to the physician as well as coordinating practical matters (van Staa, 2011). During the time of diagnosis, parents describe the importance of demonstrating strength and optimism (Young et al., 2003) and find that most parents consider informed decision-making as a fundamental part of the parental role. In an attempt to minimize their child's stress and to evade difficult conversations about the disease, parents take charge and manage the situation. However, by doing so, they also reduce opportunities for open discussions within the family, which in turn can threatening family cohesion (Phillips-Salimi et al., 2014).

Older adolescents want to be the main partners in the consultation and to avoid discussions about private matters in front of their parents (van Staa 2011). This reflects developmental theory where, even under normal circumstances, young people tend not to share private thoughts and feelings with their parents or other adults (Magni et al., 2015). Because of their increased self-identity and autonomy, adolescents viewed their parents as interfering and unnecessarily lengthening consultations (van Staa, 2011). Adolescents believe that they are 'capable of playing a more active role' but choose not to since their parents seem to take this role over or because they are bored and do not find it worthwhile (van Staa, 2011). This could be because adolescents feel that they are not listened to or taken seriously and consequently withdraw their participation. The stage of the illness and the distress levels experienced could be further limiting influences (Kelly et al., 2016). Adolescents are aware of their social positioning, relative to adults, putting them in a dependent position (Young et al., 2003) and they worry about the impact of their illness on their family and friends (Brand et al., 2017). Additionally, the concept of 'role constraints' where a patient's ability to act independently is constrained by an institution or situation, as identified by Faden and Beauchamp (1986) cited in Unguru (2011, p. 200) add to a sense of vulnerability and powerlessness as does the feeling of being excluded from discussions (Kelly et al., 2016). These constraints place them in a passive role, which through the unequal power balance, inhibits and limits their ability to participate in decision-making.

An adolescent's choice to distance themselves from the decision-making process can have varying underlying reasons and be interpreted in different ways (Clemente, 2015): reticence to communicate or take part in decisions could be because of the loss of trust in the medical profession, especially, as adolescents are more likely to experience delays in their diagnosis and have their symptoms taken less seriously (Gibson et al.2013). Adolescents may feel guilty about not recognizing their illness sooner, especially as late diagnosis is linked to poorer prognosis (Ferrari et al. 2016). During consultations leading up to their diagnosis, they need to relate the symptom history multiple times which can be frustrating and could be seen by them as a waste of time (Gibson et al 2013).

In the oncological setting, young people are mostly involved in decisions pertaining to their well-being, which has several purposes such as gaining trust, increasing compliance and giving back some control to them (Coyne et al., 2014). Compliance is rated as a significant reason for including children in the decision-making process (Wangmo et al., 2017). Adolescent inclusion in decisions, were found to be mainly non-treatment related and focused on aspects such as registration of medical data and more transient side effects such as hair loss (Wiering et al., 2016). One explanation for this could the limited treatment options available. Another reason could be and that parents and physicians implicitly attempt to convey optimism and thus focus on the immediate steps of treatment. This concentration on the short-term, together with encouragement that the adolescent is involved in non-life-threatening decisions, such as the ones regarding future fertility options, encourages participation, even if it is on a comparatively small scale.

Participation preferences vary, not only in the adolescent population but also within the individual patient throughout the course of the illness (Ruhe et al., 2015a). When adolescents are actively involved, they still seek guidance from the people they trust Weaver et al., (2015). They appreciate the role of their parents and although they value independence from their parents, they still use them as repositories for information and in the communication process as 'brokers, buffers and facilitators' (Young et al., 2003, p. 2). Parental engagement in proactive information finding and clarification is respected by ill adolescents and in fact they felt that if their parents were informed, it increased their own sense of security which in turn provided them with more confidence to participate (Weaver et al., 2015).

Although adolescents want to be able to determine their treatment, they do not want to carry full responsibility in decision-making (Coyne et al. 2014). Autonomy can be a burden and responsibility for treatment decision-making can be too overwhelming and difficult for an adolescent to make alone (Ruhe et al., 2016a) and whilst intellectually able, adolescents often lack life experience (Unguru, 2011). Especially in times of illness, children tend to trust their parents to know best (Kelly et al., 2016) at times even more than clinicians (Weaver et al., 2015). This differs greatly from the behaviour of their healthy peers (van Staa, 2011. The family unit is important to adolescents who recognize the impact their condition has on the family as a whole and as such decision-making occurs in relation to the family and ceding decisional authority to parents when necessary, is also a choice (Olzewski and Goldkind, 2018). The most supportive framework found by Weaver et al. (2015) is the integration of the patient's experience, parental support and clinicians' expertise. Coyne et al. (2014) find that for adolescents to be able to participate in decision-making in a meaningful way, they should be included according to their preferences and abilities. It is critically important to find out their preferences as often 'mere' inclusion in discourse has a higher importance than the actual decision-making process itself (Kelly et al., 2017).

With three or more parties involved in discussions, coalitions tend to build. In the medical setting this tends to be between the parents and oncologists (Gabe et al., 2004). This can lead to adolescents feeling separated from the process (Bahrami, et al. 2017) and consequently hardly contribute in triadic discussions (van Staa 2011). When physicians rely on parents as proxy-decision makers the adolescents' views may not be accurately implemented. It is crucial that adolescents are involved in discussions because their opinions and motivation can differ from that of their parents. Tulstrup et al. (2016) found that parents, in the hope of not losing their child, were more likely to enroll them in off-target drug trials whilst adolescents themselves were against further treatment. The physician facing real-life situations, and ethicist working from a theoretical stand-point view decision-making differently (Whitney et al., 2006). In order to integrate ethical considerations with pragmatic implementation, Whitney et al. (2006) developed their 'Decisional Priority in Pediatric Oncology Model' (Appendix E). They believe that under certain circumstances it is appropriate for physicians to take the lead in decision-making whilst also admitting that at times the model fails such as when parents cannot accept the fact that their child will die or conversely when the physician is unable to accept treatment failure.

Adolescents are reluctant to ask question out of embarrassment and perceived lack of physicians' time (Bahrami et al., 2017). Since adolescents often afford physicians expert status and authority, they will wait to receive information from them, rather than actively seek them out. Physicians have experience and expertise of illness and treatment and thus carry authority, power and will lead the direction of the consultations. Ideally, the professionals involved would, according to Alderson, (2007, p. 2282) be:

> "'big enough' to share information and risks, options and commitments with children, instead of trying to impose these on children."

Perceptible, limiting factors to adolescent participation in treatment decision-making exist and improvement suggestions are made in the section on links to policy and practice. First however, the main argumentation of the research findings will be discussed in the following section.

Critical Analysis

Including children and adolescents in studies is crucial to learning about their lives and perspectives in order to inform policy and provide guidelines. In the setting of paediatric cancer, a sensitive environment, respect for ethical and legal issues is crucial. Research conducted in this field tends to be limited and involves a small number of participants within the localized setting of hospitals and therefore international research articles are also included. Consequently, the findings cannot necessarily be generalized because of the small sample or culture bias but they do provide an understanding in the specific context.

Researchers have conducted studies to ascertain the viewpoints of adolescents, parents and physicians to information provision and what participation means in the treatment decision-making process. In studies with data collected from all three decision-making parties (patient, parent and physician) the associations between the different stakeholders were depicted (Bahrami et al., 2017; Wangmo et al., 2017; Essig et al., 2016; Ruhe et al., 2016b; Wiering et al., 2016). A flaw in grouping stakeholders together though, for example physicians and parents is that the perspectives of each individual group is no longer clear when grouped together as 'adults' (Wangmo et al., 2017; Ruhe et al., 2016b). In studies involving just one of the stakeholder groups, such as for adolescents (Brand et al., 2017; van Staa, 2011) or oncologists (de Vries, et al., 2010) their viewpoint remains more distinct.

As a result of the literature analysed in this review, the rationale for the necessity of adequate information provision has been demonstrated. However, perceptions on what constitutes adequate information provision differs. Adolescent cancer patients and their caregivers feel they are not adequately informed (Bahrami et al., 2017; Brand et al., 2017; Badarau et al., 2015; Clemente, 2007). Yet when Rost et al., (2017) conducted a study to find out how parents and physicians perceive information provision, they found that whilst parents found information provision to be less satisfactory physicians thought it to be adequate. Cancer survivors, from a phenomenological perspective report that insufficient information provision at diagnosis has left them with knowledge gaps in their medical history (Phillips et al., 2017; Essig et al., 2016; de Rouen et al., 2015).

For the newly diagnosed patient inadequate information provision limits their understanding of the illness, which weakens their ability to participate in their health care (Brand et al., 2017; Wangmo et al., 2017; Clemente, 2007). Inadequate information provision also leads to a loss of trust in HCPs, intensifying their isolation (Bahrami et al., 2017; Phillips et al., 2017). Physicians consider adolescents to be insufficiently competent to be involved in decision-making discussions and rely on parents as proxy decision-makers (de Vries et al., 2010). Further limiters for adolescent's participation in the treatment decision-making process are the dynamics of the family unit and parenting culture (Wangmo et al., 2017; Ruhe et al., 2016b), the nature of the illness (Day et al., 2017; Badarau et al., 2015) and the innate impulse for parents to protect their children (Wiering et al., 2016; Badarau et al., 2015; Coyne et al., 2014). Organizational constraints and physicians' regulated communication (Ruhe 2016b; Clemente 2007) add to these impacting factors. The triadic constellation of patient, parent and physician in paediatric oncology have been shown to add to the complexity of shared decision-making. Nevertheless, despite the challenges, physicians do attempt to include adolescents where possible and appropriate to the specific context (Day et al., 2017; Ruhe et al., 201a; Wiering et al., 2016). Whilst younger children are content with limited involvement, adolescents convey frustration with their limited options (Coyne et al. 2014). Having the autonomy to make treatment decisions can also be an added burden for the adolescent cancer sufferers (Ruhe et al., 2016a). Therefore, within the clinical setting, eliciting and discussing adolescents' information and decision-making preferences could improve communication (Brand et al., 2017; Day et al., 2017; Clemente, 2007) and implementing a flexible model of decision-making (Olzweski, A. and Goldkind, S., 2018; Ruhe et al., 2016a). Additionally, specialized communication training for oncologists (Essig et al., 2016; Ruhe et al., 2016b) was identified as another aspect to address the unmet information needs.

Unmistakably the adolescent patient's needs and rights to be heard are not sufficiently met. The dynamics of clinical procedure and the need to make decisions under intense pressure neither make enough provision for truly finding out how the adolescent patient wants to receive diagnostic information nor what their expectations are of their participation in treatment decision-making. Suggestions for further research in this area are made in the conclusion of this review. The links and implications for practice and policy of the research findings follow in the next section.

Links to Policy and Practice

As the diagnostic consultation is often the first time the patient and their parents meet with the physician, it is important to build rapport and trust (Coyne et al., 2014). However, because of the intense emotional turmoil the participants are under and the sense of urgency, this setting is not conducive for rational treatment decision-making. When organizing the diagnostic consultation, the following factors are important considerations to best meet the needs of all participants, particularly those of the adolescent patient.

Provision for the presence of a trusted 'other', usually parents should be made (Young et al., 2003). As not everyone is conversant with medical terms and procedures, professionals should use clear and unambiguous terms and check for understanding. Furthermore, professionals also need to listen for openings as patients may not be direct in voicing their concerns (Brand et al., 2017). Out of consideration for the preservation of normalcy and protection of other family members, patients and their parents may hide unexpressed information needs (Bluebond-Langer et al., 2005.
Consideration should also be given to the different information needs of parents who will want to be informed about treatment care and prognosis and have more long-term concerns whereas adolescents are more concerned about learning of the immediate impact their illness will have for example on appearance and on the social lives (Brand et al., 2017).
Additionally, HCPs should be cognizant of alternative sources of information seeking such as the internet if it is not provided by themselves (Essig et al., 2016).

In order to avoid misunderstanding and false assumptions at a later stage a meeting prior to the actual diagnostic consultation could take place. For example, it could take place during the time period where diagnostic tests are given and provide an opportunity to learn about the individual's sociocultural norms and individual preferences for information content and detail in anticipation of a cancer diagnosis.
When assessing ability to make decisions, a sliding scale of capacity as used for adults with cognitive impairments could be adapted for use in this scenario (Olzweski, A. and Goldkind, S., 2018). In the clinical setting, children are unlikely to disagree with a decision their parents have approved of. Therefore, a framework allowing for negotiation and shuttle diplomacy between the stakeholders, where the outcome is a collaboration could be considered (Bluebond-Langner et al. 2005). A nuanced and flexible approach to decision-making in line with adolescents' preferences may facilitate the process (Ruhe et al. 2016a).

In cases of younger adolescents, it is the physician's duty to promote the child's best interest whilst respecting the guardians' wishes. But both goals cannot always be accommodated and in times of disagreement an ethical consultation is recommended. Medical institutions employ the use of tribunals to share medical, ethical and competency decisions. To avoid therapeutic misconception, clear distinction between treatment and research is necessary, especially in this setting where the two are entwined (Woods et al., 2014).

More steps should be taken to increase awareness of young people's rights to participation concerning medical decision-making. Adolescent cancer awareness also needs to be raised. Currently the Teenage Cancer Trust, who campaign and work with MPs and Peers to improve services in the UK and are supporting a campaign to introduce cancer education awareness programmes in Scottish schools. Their campaigning is also targeted towards raising awareness for GPs to recognize adolescents' symptoms earlier and for more specialist cancer treatment units for this age group, since neither the paediatric nor adult hospitals meet their unique and specific needs.

A re-evaluation for communication training for paediatric oncologists should take place as information needs are left unmet. Best practice guidelines would include provision for adolescents to state their personal information and decisional preferences. Provision should also be made for the fact that these may change throughout the trajectory of the illness.

Conclusion

Research on the themes of adolescent cancer, communication approaches, and participation in decision-making has produced a comprehensive extended literature review and reference list. Beginning with the incidence of cancer in adolescents and the content of the diagnostic consultation followed by a discussion of the need for information and the adverse consequences of inadequate information provision. These were situated in a clinical setting to exemplify the challenges involved. The triadic shared decision-making process was examined, with attention given to the perspectives of the patient, parent and physician. The conflicted adolescent was presented in the context of the family unit and the situational difficulties they face. Under the heading of critical analysis, the main arguments were examined, and the approach taken by researchers on this topic analysed. The findings and conclusions drawn from the discussions were used to examine their implications for practice and policy.

The review concludes with a re-examination of the question, 'How do communication and information provision at diagnosis affect decision-making and participation?'. Whilst it has been shown that communication is complex and information provision substandard, affecting decision-making and participation, additional constraints for decision-making have also been identified. The review finds a conflicted adolescent, who is in transition between child and adulthood, beginning to form their own identity but through illness, is constricted: reliant on the family unit for support and encouragement and on institutionalized treatment in the hope of a cure. Decision-making cannot be measured in relation to how this age group would participate if they were healthy. Adolescents want to be informed and have honest and open communication appropriate to their needs and levels of understanding. They hold ambiguous feelings towards the responsibility of decision-making and seek support from trusted others, mostly their parents. The most important finding for the field of health care and for health care professionals is that the best interests of the adolescent are served if their information preferences are sought from the onset and a nuanced approach, based on these preferences, is applied. Only then can a young person appraise the options and make individual choices.

In furtherance to this, research on the topic of adolescent information preferences for full disclosure at diagnosis should be conducted. This could provide more information on what adolescents genuinely want to know and their expectations regarding decision-making; presently, the emphasis is still on containment and protectionism. Research which informs policy-making in clinical settings should include real-time, ethnographic studies as these more realistically reflect interaction in practice. The ethical issues concerning confidentiality, privacy and legislation surrounding research with children requires careful consideration and clinical supervision and support must be provided. In this review, the terms adolescent, young person, child(ren) were used in a generalized way to signify a group, it should be noted however, that the studies and data used in this review are based on unique and individual cases and narratives.

References

Alderson, P. (2007) `Competent children? Minors' consent to health care treatment and research', *Social science and medicine*, vol. 65, no.11, pp. 2272-2283 [Online]. Accessed 4 March 2018).

Back, A., Arnold, R., Baile, W., Tulsky, J. and Fryer-Edwards, K. (2005) `Approaching Difficult Communication Tasks in Oncology1', *CA: A Cancer journal for clinicians*, vol. 55, no. 3, pp.164-177 [Online]. (Accessed 20 March 2018).

Badarau, D. O., Wangmo, T., Ruhe, K., Miron, I., Colita, A., Dragomir, M., Schildman, J. and Elger, B. S. (2015) `Parents' challenges and physicians' tasks in disclosing cancer to children. A Qualitative interview study and reflections on professional duties in pediatric oncology', *Pediatric blood cancer*, vol. 62, pp. 2177-2182 [Online]. (Accessed 23 April 2018).

Bahrami, M., Namnabati, M., Mokarian, F., Oujian, P. and Arbon, P. (2017) `Information- sharing challenges between adolescents with cancer, their parents and health care providers: a qualitative study', *Supportive care in cancer: official journal of the multinational association of supportive care in cancer*, vol. 25, no. 5, pp.1587-1596 [Online]. (Access 12 April 2018)

Bleyer, A., Ferrari, A., Whelan, J., & Barr, R. (2017) `Global assessment of cancer incidence and survival in adolescents and young adults', *Pediatric blood and cancer*, vol. 64 no. 9, [Online]. (Accessed 15 March 2018).

Bluebond-Langer, M. (2005) 'Involving children with life-shortening illnesses in decisions about participation in clinical research: a proposal for shuttle diplomacy and negotiation' pp. 323-343 in Smith, R. C. and Kodish, E. (eds) *Ethics and research with children: A case-based approach*. Oxford; New York: Oxford University Press [Online]. (Accessed 27 April 2018).

Bosco, F.M., and Angeleri, R. (2010) `Communication' in Cummings, L. (ed.) *The pragmatics encyclopedia* London: Routledge [Online]. (Accessed 26 March 2018).

Brand, S., Fasciano, K., and Mack, J. (2017) `Communication preferences of pediatric cancer patients: talking about prognosis and their future life', *Supportive care in cancer*, vol. 25, no. 3, pp. 769-774 [Online]. (Accessed 22 April 2018).

Clemente, I. (2007) `Clinicians' routine use of non- disclosure: prioritizing "protection" over the information needs of adolescents with cancer', *Canadian journal of nursing research*, vol. 39 no. 4, pp. 19-34 [Online].
(Accessed 22 April 2018).

Clemente, I. (2015) *Uncertain futures: communication and culture in childhood cancer treatment*. Chichester, Wiley Blackwell.

Coulter, A. and Collins, A. (2011) *Making Shared Decision-Making a Reality: No decision about me, without me*. Kings Fund Report. London [Online].
(Accessed 30 March 2018).

Coyne, I., Amory, A., Kiernan, G. and Gibson, F. (2014) `Children's participation in shared decision-making: children, adolescents, parents and healthcare professionals' perspectives and experiences' *European journal of oncology nursing*, vol. 18, no. 3, pp. 273-280 [Online]. (Accessed 28 March 2018).

Coyne I, O'Mathúna DP, Gibson F, Shields L, Leclercq E, Sheaf G. (2016) `Interventions for promoting participation in shared decision-making for children with cancer', *Cochrane Database of Systematic Reviews*, issue 11, art. no.: CD008970 [Online]. (Accessed 21 February 2018).

Day, E., Jones, L., Langner, R., Stirling, L. C., Hough, R., & Bluebond-Langner, M. (2017) "We just follow the patients' lead": Healthcare professional perspectives on the involvement of teenagers with cancer in decision making'. *Pediatric blood and cancer*, vol. 65, no. 3, [Online]. (Accessed 22 April 2018).

Dekking, S. A. S., van der Graaf, R., Kars, M. C., Beishuizen, A., de Vries, M. and van Delden, J. J. M. (2015) `Balancing research interests and patient interests: a qualitative study into the intertwinement of care research in paediatric oncology', *Pediatric blood cancer*, vol. 62, pp. 816-822 [Online].
(Accessed 1 March 2018).

De Clercq, E., Ruhe, K., Rost, M. and B. Elger (2017) `Is decision-making capacity an "essentially contested"concept in pediatrics?' Medicine, health care and philosophy, vol. 20, no. 3, pp. 425-433 [Online]. (Accessed 9 April 2018).

De Rouen, M. C., Smith, A. W., Tao, L., Bellizzi, K. M., Lynch, C. F., Parsons, H. M., Kent, E. E. and Keegan, T. H. M. (2015) `Cancer-related information needs and cancer's impact on control over life influence health- related quality of life among adolescents and young adults with cancer: Information needs and control influence HRQOL among AYA cancer survivors', Psycho-oncology, vol. 24, no. 9, pp. 1104-1115 [Online]. (Accessed 21 March 2018).

De Vries, M. C., Wit, J. M., Engberts, D. P., Kaspers, G. J. L. and van Leeuwen, E. (2010) `Pediatric oncologists' attitudes towards involving adolescents in decision-making concerning research participation', Pediatric blood cancer, vol. 55, no. 1, pp. 123-128 [Online]. Available at (Accessed 29 March 2018).

De Vries, M., Houtlosser, M., Wit, J. M., Engberts, D.P., Bresters, D., Kaspers, G.JL. and van Leeuwen, E. (2011) `Ethical issues at the interface of clinical care and research in pediatric oncology: a narrative review of parents' and physicians' experiences', BMC medical ethics, vol.12, pp. 18-18 [Online]. (Accessed 21 March 2018).

Essig, S., Steiner, C., Kuehni, C. E., Weber, H. and Kiss, A. (2016) `Improving communication in adolescent cancer care: a multi-perspective study', Pediatric blood and cancer, vol. 63, no. 8, pp.1423-1430 [Online]. (Accessed 22 April 2018).

Ferrari, A., Lo Vullo, S., Giardiello, D., Veneroni, L., Magni, C., Clerici, C. A., Chiaravalli, S., Casanova, M., Luksch, R., Terenzianai, M., Spreafico, F., Meazza, C., Catania, S., Schiavello, E., Biassoni, V., Podda, M., Bergamaschi, L., Puma, N., Massimino, M. and Mariani, L. (2016) `The sooner the better? How symptom interval correlates with outcome in children and adolescents with solid tumors: regression tree analysis of the findings of a prospective study', Pediatric blood and cancer, vol. 63, no. 3, pp. 479-485 [Online]. (Accessed 14 February 2018).

Gabe, J., Olumide, G., an Bury, M. (2004) ```It takes three to tango": a framework for understanding patient partnership in paediatric clinics', *Social science and medicine*, vol. 59, no. 5, pp. 1071-1079 [Online]. (Accessed 17 March 2018).

Gibson, F., Pearce, S., Eden, T., Glaser, A., Hooker, L., Whelan, J., and Kelly, D. (2013) `Young people describe their pre-diagnosis cancer experience', *Psycho-oncology*, vol. 22, no. 11, pp. 2585-2592 [Online].
(Accessed 18 March 2018).

Graham, A. and Fitzgerald, R (2010) `Children's participation in research: some possibilities and constraints in the current Australian research environment', *Journal of sociology*, vol. 46, no. 2, pp. 133-147 [Online].
(Accessed 8 April 18).

Hein, I. M., Troost, P. W., Broersma, A., de Vries, M. C., Daams, J. G., and Lindauer, R. J. L. (2015) 'Why is it hard to make progress in assessing children's decision-making competence?', *BMC medical ethics*, vol. 16, no. 1 [Online]. (Accessed 31 March 2018).

Ilowite, M. F., Cronin, A. M., Kang, T. I., and Mack, J. W. (2017) `Disparities in prognosis communication among parents of children with cancer: the impact of race and ethnicity', *Cancer*, vol. 123, no. 20, pp. 3995-4003 [Online]. (Accessed 7 March 2018).

Kelly, K., Mowbray, C., Pyke-Grimm, K. and Hinds, P. S. (2016) `Identifying a conceptual shift in child and adolescent-reported treatment decision making: "Having a say, as I need at this time"', *Pediatric blood and cancer*,
vol. 64, no. 4 [Online]. (Accessed 16 April 2018).

Kessel, R. M., Roth, M., Moody, K. and Levy, A. (2013) `Day one talk: parent preferences when learning that their child has cancer', *Supportive care in cancer*, vol. 21, no. 11, pp. 2977-2982 [Online]. (Accessed 19 February 2018).

Kilicarslan-Toruner, E., and Akgun-Citak, E. (2012) `Information seeking behaviors and decision-making process of parents of children with cancer', *European journal of oncology nursing*, Manuscript [Online]. (Accessed 1 April 2018).

Korsvold, L., Lie, H. C., Mellblom, A. V., Ruud, E., Loge, J. H. and Finset, A. (2016a) `Tailoring the delivery of cancer diagnosis to adolescent and young adult patients displaying strong emotions: An observational study of two cases'. *International journal of qualitative studies on health and well-being*, vol. 11, no. 1 [Online]. (Accessed 16 April 2018).

Korsvold, L., Mellblom, A. V., Lie, H. C., Ruud, E., Loge, J. H., and Finset, A. (2016b) `Patient-provider communication about the emotional cues and concerns of adolescent and young adult patients and their family members when receiving a diagnosis of cancer', *Patient education and counseling*, vol. 99, no. 10, pp. 1576-1583 [Online]. (Accessed 22 March 2018).

Mack, J. W. and Joffe., S., (2014) `Communicating about prognosis: ethical responsibilities of pediatricians and parents', *Pediatrics*. vol. 133, no. 2, pp. 24-30 [Online]. (Accessed 13 March 2018).

Magni, M. C., Veneroni, L., Clerici, C. A., Proserpio, T., Sironi, G., Casanova, M., Chiaravalli, S., Massimino, M. and Ferrari, A. (2015) `New strategies to ensure good patient-physician communication when treating adolescents and young adults with cancer: the proposed model of the Milan Youth Project', *Clinical oncology in adolescents and young adults,* vol. 5, no. 63, pp. 63-73 [Online]. (Accessed 13 March 2018).

Nuffield Council of Bioethics, (2017) *Children and clinical research: ethical issues*, Nuffield Council on Bioethics, London [Online]. (Accessed 11 April 2018).

Olson, R., Bobinski, M. A., Ho, A. and Goddard, K. (2012) `Oncologists' view of informed consent and shared decision making in paediatric radiation oncology', *Radiotherapy and oncology*, vol. 102, no. 2, pp. 210-213 [Online]. (Accessed 11 March 2018).

Olzweski, A. and Goldkind, S. (2018) 'The default position: optimising pediatric participation in medical decision making', *The American journal of bioethics*, vol. 18, no. 3, pp. 4-9 [Online]. (Accessed 21 April 2018.

Phillips, R. C., Haase, E. J., Broome, E. M., Carpenter, S. J. and Frankel, M. R. (2017) `Connecting with healthcare providers at diagnosis: adolescent/young adult cancer survivors? perspectives'. International journal of qualitative studies on health and well-being, vol. 12, no. 1 [Online]. (Accessed 11 April 2012).

Phillips-Salimi, C. R., Robb, S. L., Monahan, P. O., Doessey, A. and Haase, J. E. (2014) `Perceptions of communication, family adaptability and cohesion: a comparison of adolescents newly diagnosed with cancer and their parents', *International journal of adolescent medical health*, vol. 26, no.1, pp. 19-26 [Online]. (Accessed 27 February 2018).

Rost, M., Wangmo, T., Niggli, F., Hartmann, K., Hengartner, H., Ansari, M., Brazzola, P., Rischewski, J., Beck-Popovic, M., Kühne, T. and Elger, B. (2017) `Parents' and physicians' perceptions of children's participation in decision-making in paediatric oncology: a quantitative study, *Journal of bioethical inquiry*, vol. 14, no. 4, pp. 556-565 [Online]. (Accessed 22 April 2018)

Ruhe, K. M., Badarau, D. O., Brazzola, P., Hengartner, H., Elger, B. S., and Wangmo, T. (2016a) `Participation in pediatric oncology: views of child and adolescent patients', *Psycho-oncology*, vol. 25, no. 9, pp. 1036-1042 [Online]. (Accessed 10 April 2018).

Ruhe, K., Wangmo, T., De Clercq, E., Badarau, D., Ansari, M., Kühne, T., Niggli, F. and Elger, B. (2016b) `Putting patient participation into practice in pediatrics - results from a qualitative study in pediatric oncology. *European journal of pediatrics*, vol.175, no. 9, pp. 1147-1155 [Online]. (Accessed 12 April 2018).

Steinberg, L. (2013) `Does recent research on adolescent brain development inform the mature minor doctrine?', *Journal of medicine and philosophy*, vol. 38, no. 3, pp. 256-267 [Online]. (Accessed 2 March 2018).

Streuli, J. C., Michel, M., and Vayena, E. (2011) `Children's rights in pediatrics', *European journal of pediatrics*, vol. 170, no. 1, pp. 9-14 [Online]. (Accessed 20 February 2018).

Talati, E. D., Lang, C. W. and Ross, L. F. (2010) `Reactions of pediatricians to refusals of medical treatment for minors', *Journal of adolescent health*, vol. 47, no. 2, pp. 126-132 [Online]. (Accessed 28 February 2018).

Teenage Cancer Trust (2016) *The blue print of cancer care for teenagers and young adults with cancer. 2nd ed.* Edited by Smith, E., Mooney, S., Cable, M. and Taylor, R. M [Online]. (Accessed on 4 March 2018).

Thompson, K., Dyson, G., Holland, L., and Joubert, L. (2013) `An exploratory study of oncology specialists' understanding of the preferences of young people living with cancer', *Social work in health care*, vol. 52, no. 2-3, pp.166-190 [Online]. (Accessed 20 March 2018).

Tulstrup, M., Larsen, H. B., Castor, A., Rossel, P., Grell, K., Heyman, M., Abrahamsson, J., Söderhäll, S., Asberg, A., Jonsson, O. G., Vettenranta, K., Frandsen, T. L., Albertsen, B. and Schmiegelow, K. (2016) `Parents' and adolescents' preferences for intensified or reduced treatment in randomized lymphoblastic leukemia trials', *Pediatric blood and cancer*, vol. 63, no. 5, pp. 865-871[Online]. (Accessed 28 February 2018).

Twamley, K., Craig, F., Kelly, P., Hollowell, D. R., Mendoza, P., and Bluebond-Langner, M. (2014) `Underlying barriers to referral to paediatric palliative care services', *Journal of child health care*, vol. 18, no. 1, pp.19-30 [Online]. (Accessed 2 February 2018).

Unguru, Y. (2011) `Making sense of adolescent decision-making: challenge and reality', in *Ethical and legal issues in adolescent health care: STARs ethical and legal Issues in adolescent health care*, vol. 22, no. 2, pp. 195-206 in Silber, T. J. and English, A. (eds) American Academy of Pediatrics, ProQuest Ebook Central, [Online]. (Accessed 26 March 2018).

United Nation Human Rights Office of the High Commissioner (1990). *Convention on the Rights of the Child* [Online]. (Accessed 30 December 2017).

Van Staa, A. (2011) `Unraveling triadic communication in hospital consultations with adolescents with chronic conditions: The added value of mixed methods research', *Patient education and counseling*, vol. 82, no. 3, pp, 455-464 [Online]. (Accessed 16 April 2018).

Vetsch, J., Fardell, J. E., Wakefield, C. E., Signorelli, C., Michel, G., McLoone, J. K., Walwyn, T., Tapp, H., Truscott, J. and Cohn, R. J. (2017) `"Forewarned and forearmed": Long- term childhood cancer survivors' and parents' information needs and implications for survivorship models of care', *Patient education and counseling*, vol. 100, no. 2, pp. 355-363 [Online]. (Accessed 13 February 2018).

Wangmo, T., De Clercq, E., Ruhe, K. M., Beck-Popovic, M., Rischewski, J., Angst, R., Ansari, M., and Elger, B. S. (2017) `Better to know than to imagine: Including children in their health care', *AJOB Empirical Bioethics*, vol. 8, no. 1, pp. 11-20 [Online]. (Accessed 28 February 2018).

Weaver, M. S., Baker, J. N., Gattuso, J. S., Gibson, D. V., Sykes, A. D. and Hinds, P. S. (2015) `Adolescents' preferences for treatment decisional involvement during their cancer', *Cancer*, vol. 121, no. 24, pp. 4416-4424 [Online]. (Accessed 13 April 2018).

Whitney, S. N., Ethier, A. M., Frugé, E., Berg, S., McCullough, L. B. and Hockenberry, M. (2006) `Decision making in pediatric oncology: who should take the lead? The decisional priority in pediatric oncology model', *Journal of clinical oncology,* vol. 24, no. 1, pp. 160-165 [Online]. (Accessed on 27 March 2018).

Wiener, L., Weaver, M. S., Bell, C. J., and Sansom-Daly, U. M. (2015) `Threading the cloak: palliative care education for care providers of adolescents and young adults with cancer', *Clinical oncology in adolescents and young adults*, vol. 5, no. 1, pp. 1-18 [Online]. (Accessed 27 March 2018).

Wiering, B. M., Noordman, J., Tates, K., Zwaanswijk, M., Elwyn, G., de Bont, E. S. J. M., Beishuizen, A., Hoogerbrugge, P.M. and van Dulmen, S. (2016) `Sharing decisions during diagnostic consultations; an observational study in pediatric oncology', *Patient education and counseling*, vol.99, no. 1, pp. 61-67 [Online]. (Accessed 22 April 2018).

Woods, S., Hagger, L., and McCormack, P. (2014) `Therapeutic misconception: Hope, trust and misconception in paediatric research', *Health care analysis*, vol. 22, no. 1, pp. 3-21 [Online]. (Accessed 2 March 2018).

Yeomanson, D. J., Morgan, S., and Pacey, A. A. (2013) `Discussing fertility preservation at the time of cancer diagnosis: dissatisfaction of young females', *Pediatric blood and cancer*, vol. 60, no. 12, pp. 1996-2000 [Online].
(Accessed 1 March 2018).

Young, B., Dixon-Woods, M., Windridge, K. C. and Heney, D. (2003) `Managing communication with young people who have a potentially life- threatening chronic illness: qualitative study of patients and parents', *British Medical Journal*, vol. 326, pp. 305-308 [Online]. (Accessed 2 April 2018).

Appendices

Appendix A

The following three excerpts indicate the increasing incidence of cancer in adolescents and young adults and are copied directly from Bleyer et al. (2017, p. 4).

Excerpt 1: A bullet point list, highlighting the increasing incidence of cancer in adolescents and young adults, copied from Bleyer et al. (2017, p. 3).

Highlights

- More than a million new diagnoses of cancer are made annually among a global population of 3 billion AYAs worldwide.

- The global burden of cancer in AYAs is higher than in all other age groups.

- The overall incidence of invasive cancer among AYAs in high-income countries has been increasing among AYAs.

- In the United States, the rate of increase since 1975 has been higher than in any other age group, the magnitude of which has persisted since 1990 when all age groups above 55 have had a decrease.

- Since 1990, when the incidence began decreasing in Americans over age 55, AYAs had even greater relative increase in the incidence of cancer that was particularly evident in females.

Excerpt 2: Bar chart copied from Bleyer et al. (2017, p. 4).

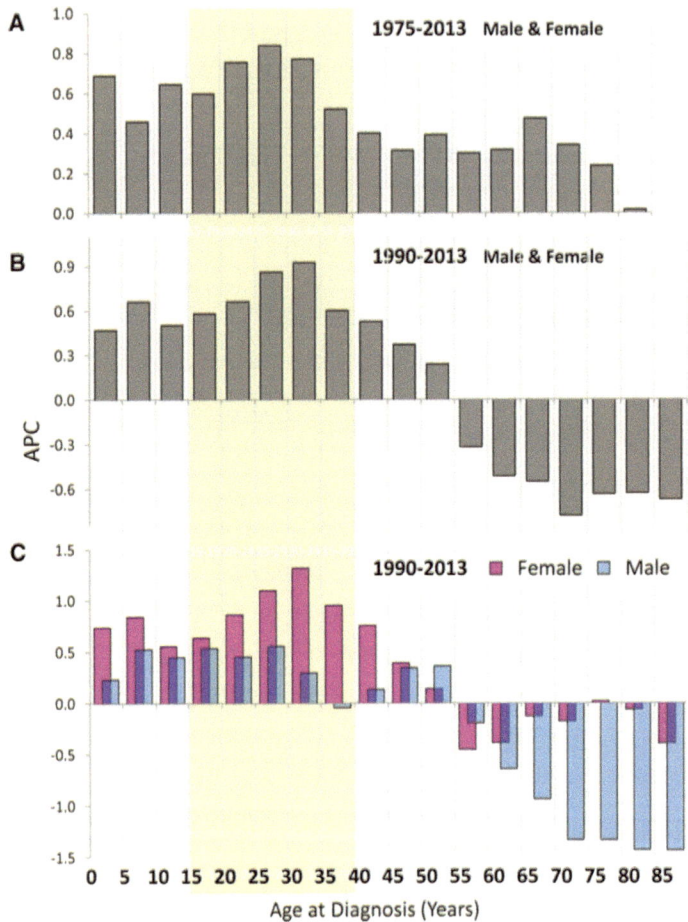

FIGURE 2 Average APC in incidence of all invasive cancer except KS in males, 1975–2013 (A), 1990–2013 (B and C) and 1990–2013 by sex (C), United States SEER 9 regions

Excerpt 3: Graphs copied from Bleyer et al. (2017, p. 4).

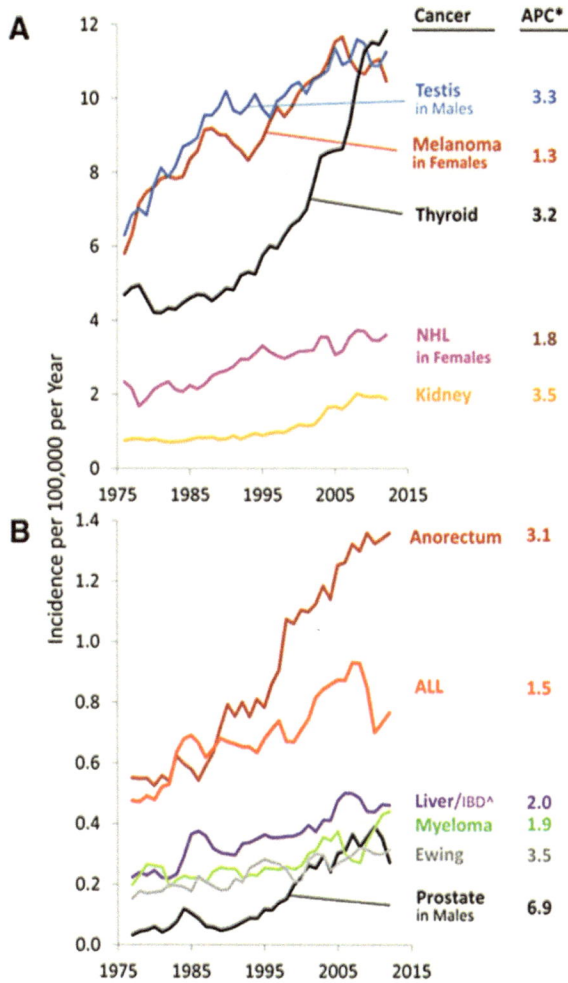

FIGURE 3 Annual incidence of cancers in AYAs that increased in incidence during 1975–2012, United States SEER 9 regions. Curves (A) are 2-year moving averages and curves (B) are 3-year moving averages. *APC: annual percent change during 1975–2012, all values of which are statistically significant at P values less than 10^−9. ^Anal: anal cancer, anorectum and rectal cancer combined. †Intrahepatic bile duct

Appendix B

The disparity between what is important to adolescents and what HCPs perceive is of importance to them copied from Thompson et al. (2013 p.172).

TABLE 2 Health Care Professionals' Perceptions of the Five Most Salient Issues for AYA Living With Cancer and the Most Salient Issues Reported by Young People

Top five broad health care issues for AYA living with cancer	Perceived top five issues for AYA living with cancer by health care professionals
1 Maintaining engagement in school, education, & employment	1 Survival of a cancer diagnosis
2 Changes to relationships: Family, partners, peers	2 Relapse, dying, the future
3 Fertility & sexual well-being including body image & self-identity	3 Functional well-being/Loss of independence impacted by treatment side effects
4 Provision of accurate information to assist in knowledge development and informed decision making	4 Relationships: Family, partners, peers
5 Inadequate hospital facilities and unsuitable hospital environment	5 Fertility and future prospects for parenthood

Appendix C

A case study of the diagnostic consultation related by a patient and their family[1]

Present at the diagnostic consultation: Dr. F.*, Dr. M.*, Ms. H*, adolescent patient, father and mother

Dr. M.* opens the meeting informing us that he is a surgeon. He tells them the tumour, an osteosarcoma, is very aggressive, malignant, rare and that it can be cured in 70% of cases. He informs them that the treatment will involve chemotherapy before and after surgery. Without a discussion he states that they are going to follow a curative path and that this inter-disciplinary sarcoma centre with its team of specialists, is the best equipped to treat the patient.

Dr. F.* introduces himself and his function as oncologist. He states that whereas he agrees with his colleague on all the points described he feels that he needs to correct Dr. M.* on one point which is that realistically the chances of cure were closer to 60%. He explains the expected time frame involved and some of the lesser side-effects of chemotherapy.

Ms. H.* explains her function as case manager and the most immediate procedures which will need to take place over the next few days such as pre-treatment check-ups and the implant of a port-a-cath.

The adolescent patient, father and mother stay in the consulting room after the staff leave and are thus given the opportunity to express suppressed emotions before leaving the hospital themselves.

At the end of the diagnostic consultation, the patient and their family believe:

- *Patient could be cured both because a curative treatment plan has been prescribed and because no alternative option has been provided.*
- *That the patient and the family will be kept informed and involved in the treatment decision-making process.*
- *That the treating hospital is a specialised sarcoma centre, with the different departments involved (orthopaedics, pathology and oncology) working together.*
- *Dr. M.* is a surgeon specialising in sarcomas.*
- *Ms. H* will act as co-ordinator for organising the upcoming procedures and will function as an interface between us and the physicians.*

The patient and family are not told about alternative treatment options or the inclusion of palliative care services and do not have the where-with-all to consider what the alternatives might be as they are traumatized and in shock.

During the consultation they had not been provided with information on:

---

[1] The family is known to the author

- The sub-type of osteosarcoma and when they subsequently enquired about it, were told it was irrelevant (which is incorrect as the sub-type is a predictor of chemotherapy efficacy).
- The stage of the disease.
- The more severe side-effects of chemotherapy.
- Other sarcoma centres existing in the country and were therefore left with the impression that this centre was the only option to treat the osteosarcoma.

After the treatment had started, they learnt that:

- Patient's chances of cure were much lower than they were told, based on the size of the tumour on presentation and its location.
- There did not appear to be a rehabilitation plan in place after treatment despite the emphasis on cure.

Clearly, the physicians had dictated a course of treatment without providing the patient and their family with the full facts. This raises ethical issues concerning informed consent.

Once the patient was caught in the system, they also found that the term 'inter-disciplinary sarcoma centre' and the portrayal of the disciplines working closely and professionally together as described to them at diagnosis, did not meet the reality they experienced.

- In practice they evidenced: lacking co-ordination, miscommunication and non-communication within the respective disciplines, with the other departments involved and with the patient and their family themselves. In fact, they found that it was a constant battle to obtain fact-based information throughout the illness trajectory, requiring energy and tenacity.
- They were misinformed and disinformed about: treatment options, disease progression and further treatment options.
- Whilst Ms. H.* would co-ordinate appointments, she would not act as case manager in the way that they were led to believe she would. In order to gain information, it was necessary for the patient and/or their family to contact each discipline involved separately.

*Whilst the real names of those involved are not used here in order to protect their anonymity, they are known to the author.

Appendix D

A sample of potential questions which physicians could use to elicit adolescent patient views directly linked to the most relevant articles UNCRC (1989), directly copied from Streuli et al., (2011, p. 13).

Table 3 Practical implications of the UNCRC

Deduced questions (related article)

Do I try my best to arrange all conversations with children and parents undisturbed in a likable atmosphere with sufficient time? (Art. 3, 9, 16, 23, 31)

Do I rather talk with the child than only about the child as soon as possible? (Art. 12, 13, 16)

Do I explain the whole purpose of a treatment or an intervention to the child in an age-appropriate manner? [duration, speed, pauses, word choice, demonstration with drawings, toys, videos or computer] (Art. 12, 13, 30, 31)

Do I indicate to the child that he or she can know everything, even if it could be difficult to understand everything? (Art. 13)

Does the child have enough time and support for a proper decision making process? Are there repeated opportunities to raise questions? (Art. 5, 13, 31)

Do I let the child feel that it would not be alone with his or her problems? (Art. 9, 19, 24)

Am I of sufficient openness and impartiality for a proper dialog? (Art. 2, 12, 13)

Does the child with linguistic and/or symbolic communication make a contribution to the decision making process? (Art. 3, 12)

Do I try to understand arguments and decisions even if they seem wrong to me? Do I appreciate the cultural background as a part of the child's interests? (Art. 12, 24, 27, 22, 30)

Do we determine the child's best interests interdisciplinarily by a broader consultation including children and parents or merely from the biomedical perspective? (Art. 3, 5, 9, 18, 24, 31)

Do I allow the child to acquire experience with the decision making process in well-considered and appropriate situations, and in such cases do I even allow the child to make the wrong decisions? (Art. 6, 12, 13, 30)

Do I provide and plan with the same professionalism curative as well as supportive, palliative, and comfort therapy? (Art. 3, 19, 23)

Do I take into consideration the basic needs of the child and his or her family? (Art. 6, 18, 19, 22, 27)

Do I advance my communication skills through appropriate training? (Art. 2, 3, 6, 12, 13, 24)

Appendix E

The Decisional Priority in Pediatric Oncology Model

The model illustrates the complexity involved in pediatric oncology decision-making. The components of the model are a continuum of: possibility of cure, treatment options and decisional priority.

(Whitney et al. 2006, p. 162)

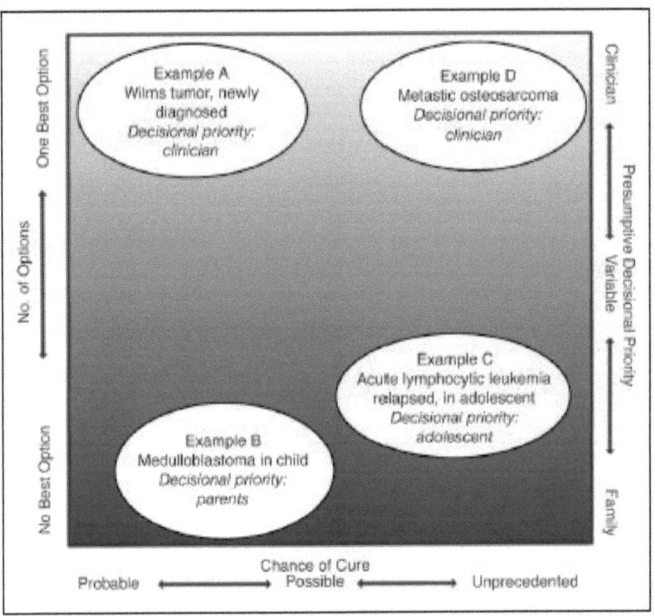

Based on the examples above, in example A there is a good chance of curing the disease but there is only one form of treatment, and therefore the clinician makes the treatment decision because there is little choice for the family. In the case of example B, again the treatment is curative, but there are different treatment options available, whereby the family make the ultimate choice, based on information from the clinician. In example C, the prognosis is poor and the options the family faces are palliative care or participation in drug trials. In contrast, example D, although the prognosis is poor, there is still a standard treatment option, which the clinician decides is the best option.

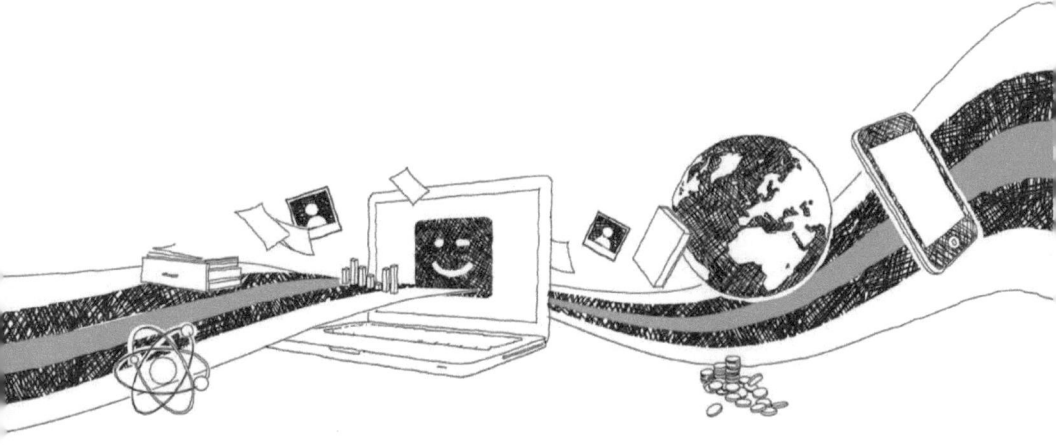
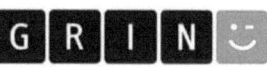